THE ULTIMATE MEDITERRANEAN DIET COOKBOOK #2020

Lose Weight with Easy and Nutritious Recipes incl. 28 Days Weight Loss Plan

MARC J. WILLIAMS

ISBN - 9798684944352

TABLE OF CONTENTS

WHAT IS THE MEDITERRANEAN DIET?

One of the most popular diets in recent times is the Mediterranean diet. This was attributed to the fact that it was voted as one of the most popular diets of the year 2019. The main reason was the numerous exciting possibilities it offers and the many individuals jumping on its train.

Lots of research have been carried out with regard to this, and many benefits such as weight loss, heart health, and an improved brain function have been outlined. The Mediterranean diet plan is all about lifestyle rather than the food itself. It is solely based on how the people in the Mediterranean region eat and prepare their meals.

In its entirety, there is no definitive guide to the diet. In other words, there cannot be a way to fully spell out what to eat, how to eat, and when to eat. Instead, you are more likely to find a wide array of recipes, guidelines, and cookbooks all dedicated to showing you how to fully tap into the many benefits Mediterranean diets have to offer, in different ways.

WHY SHOULD YOU GO FOR THE DIET?

As far back as the 60s, there have been increased observations that coronary heart disease wreaked the least havoc in the Mediterranean nation-states. Countries such as Italy, particularly southern Italy, Crete, and Greece had fewer deaths than countries in northern Europe and the U.S. Other studies carried out also showed that the diet is linked with reduced risk factors of cardiovascular disease.

The world health organization, UNESCO, and other figures in the American wellness industry have recommended the Mediterranean meal plan is ideal for promoting health. It is fully recognized as a sustainable and healthy dietary plan you can tap into. The diet is widely recognized as an intangible cultural asset.

The Mediterranean diet consists solely of the region's traditional meals and fruits, and all the cooking methods. It is vegetables, nuts, seafood, dairy, and olive oil. To spice things up, one or two glasses of wine can also be included for premium enjoyment. Get those endorphins pumping!

WHAT IS THE MEDITERRANEAN DIET COMPOSED OF?

Although there is no single definition for the Mediterranean diet, there is no complete description of what it essentially entails. However, from earlier descriptions, it is a diet that contains a high proportion of the following major components:

✓ Weekly intake of poultry, beans, fish, and eggs.

✓ Daily consumption of whole grains, healthy fats, fruits, and vegetables.

✓ Reasonable amounts of dairy products.

✓ Limited intake of red meat.

There are also some other inclusions such as a glass of wine after the meal, sharing the meal itself with family and close friends, all in a bid to improve mental health, and be physically active. At this point, it is prudent that we highlight the important parts of the Mediterranean diet as a whole.

Healthy Fats

Healthy fats are consumed as alternatives to trans and saturated fats which increases the risk of developing heart disease. Olive oil is considered a good primary source of fat in the Mediterranean diet. It provides monounsaturated fat which contributes to overall health by lowering body cholesterol level, bad lipoproteins, and low-density lipoprotein.

The nuts and seeds which are a part of the diet also contain monounsaturated fats. Fatty fishes like sardines, salmon, lake trout, herring, and albacore tuna are said to be rich in omega-3 fatty acids.

What of the wine?

While some may have exceptions to the inclusion of red wine in the Mediterranean diet, it allows the drinking of wine in moderation. The dietary guidelines for Americans however, warn against drinking it in excess. It advises on properly weighing the risk to benefit ratio before deciding if it is safe to drink. The moderate amounts of wine allowed mean nothing less than 5oz for women and no more than 10oz daily for men (Approx. 2 glasses).

HOW DOES THE MEDITERRANEAN DIET WORK?

The Mediterranean diet isn't inclined to help achieve weight loss. This does not also mean it is lost on providing the benefit of helping to achieve a reduction in weight. At least out of the wide array of dieting plans available, the Mediterranean diet was ranked the top ten amongst weight-loss diets.

It was not essentially built like a weight loss plan, but it has managed to gain popularity due to its all-encompassing approach to eating, unlike the other diets. Two out of the five blue zones where people are known to live longer due to lower rates of diseases and overall healthier meals are in Mediterranean cities.

The Mediterranean diet harps on eating vegetables, fruits, whole grains, nuts, beans, legumes, olive oil, spices, and flavorful herbs. The inclusion of seafood and fish a few times a week; Cheese, eggs, poultry, and yogurt consumption in moderation is also advised, while still saving wine, sweets, and red meat. Red wine contains resveratrol which is a compound known among the locals to add more years to life.

WILL THE MEDITERRANEAN DIET HELP YOU TO LOSE WEIGHT?

Many fear that eating foods that make up the Mediterranean diet which is rich in fats, olives, cheese, and avocado is sure to keep them fat. However, more and more research done over time is suggesting that the opposite is true.

This to an extent, depends on the aspects of the diet you adopt and how that compares to your current meal plan. For example, it is advised that to build a calorie-deficit meal into your plan you need to eat fewer calories than the daily recommended amount and complement by burning off extra amounts through exercises to help you shed more pounds.

MYTHS ABOUT THE MEDITERRANEAN DIET:

The diet is only about Food:

Many are quick to think the diet is solely about the food while leaving the other parts of the diet, such as the physical activities and the general way of living. When people in the region sit down in a relaxed mood for a good meal, as opposed to sitting in front of a television when eating or not eating in a rushed manner in any way.

It is expensive to eat this way:

Some are of the opinion that the Mediterranean diet is very expensive. But think of it this way, if you are solely feeding on a meal mainly composed of lentils or beans as a main source of protein; while supplementing with vegetables and whole grains, then the diet is way less expensive than consuming dishes of processed and packaged foods.

Filling yourself up with bowls of pasta and bread is the ideal Mediterranean Way:

Contrary to what many think, folks in the Mediterranean do not consume big bowls of pasta unlike Americans do. Alternatively, they prefer to reserve pasta as a side dish with minimal servings. Either a cup or half-cup serving size. The rest of the plate contains fish, organic, grass-fed meat, vegetables, salad, and maybe a slice of bread.

HOW MUCH DOES THE DIET ACTUALLY COST?

When it comes to the cost of the Mediterranean diet, and just like all aspects of the diet, the cost depends on how you shape it. Although in some localities, the essentials of the diet like olive oil, fresh vegetable produce, fish, and nuts can be expensive, there is a way you can keep the tab relatively within your means.

If you are replacing the red meats in your diet with plant-based home cooking meals, you are more likely to cut down on costs. Shopping choices have an effect too. If you cannot get a bottle of wine for about $50, you can decide to get another for $15, and you can just get whatever veggies are for sale that day, instead of having to spend about $3 on the artichokes.

HEALTH BENEFITS OF THE MEDITERRANEAN DIET:

Preventing heart diseases and stroke

This should not be surprising in any way. The Mediterranean diet restricts the intake of processed foods, red meat, refined slices of bread and encourages the drinking of red wine in moderation instead of drowning cups of hard liquor. These are all factors that can reduce the risk of you developing stroke and heart disease.

Reducing the risk of Alzheimer's

Research conducted into unraveling the benefits of Mediterranean diets has revealed that it helps to improve blood sugar levels, cholesterol, and maintain optimum blood vessel health. This will in turn reduce the risk of developing dementia or Alzheimer's disease.

Reducing the risk of Parkinson's disease

The high proportion of antioxidants in Mediterranean diets, gotten from the high proportion of vegetables, and fruits helps to prevent cells from undergoing the process of oxidative stress. This cuts the risk of developing Parkinson's disease in half.

For agility

Coupled with the physical activity advised as an integral of the Mediterranean diet, if you are an older adult, the nutrients derived from the diet goes a long way in reducing the risk of you developing muscle weakness and other obvious signs of frailty by as far as 70%.

Protection against type 2 diabetes

This may come as a surprise since there is the general mythical knowledge that any diet rich in sugar or sugar-like items such as the wine regarded as an integral of this diet, amongst other things cannot be seen to help in protection against type 2 diabetes.

However, this is an exception. The Mediterranean diet is very rich in fiber and digests slowly. It helps to prevent swings in blood sugar and also goes a long way in maintaining a healthy weight.

DOWNSIDES OF THE DIET INCLUDE

A major con of the Mediterranean diet is its stance on the consumption of milk. Milk is limited and if you are that guy who loves drinking milk, you might have to stay off it and in return get your calcium supply from eating yogurt and cheese. You can also consider drinking skim milk.

You need to always find time to cook

Due to the need for delicious fresh food now and then on the diet, one learning curve you might experience on the Mediterranean diet is the fact that you will have to spend hours in your kitchen cooking. If you are the type that does not love cooking, then maybe you might need to make another choice on your preferred meal plan.

A detailed and all-encompassing Mediterranean diet cookbook is not complete without the list of the foods to eat and those to avoid when you choose to latch onto the many benefits this diet offers. This list has nutritional stats attached to them for improved understanding.

RECOMMENDED FOOD WHILE ON THE DIET

Salmon

Fish like salmon is allowed on the Mediterranean diet. It is a rich source of omega-3-fatty acids. The American Heart Association recommends eating at least two fish containing meals per week, particularly one containing rich and beneficial fats like Salmon.

Tomatoes

Tomatoes are fully packed with lycopene which is a highly beneficial antioxidant associated with a reduced risk of certain cancers such as the cancer of the breast and prostate. There are some other components in tomatoes that help to reduce the risk of developing sudden blood clots thereby strengthening your body against cardiovascular disease.

Olive oil

This another beneficial and at the same time essential component of the Mediterranean diet. One of the major differences the diet has when compared to other meal plans is the fact that it has replaced foods high in saturated fats like butter with plant sources rich in monounsaturated fatty; acids, an example being olive oil.

Chickpeas

The main nutrition in chickpeas, hummus contains a sizable amount of fiber, coupled with lots of zinc, iron, folate, and magnesium. Which according to a paper published in November 2014 in the Journal of applied nutrition, metabolism and physiology. The statistics available are for a whole cup and you only need just half a cup to reap the benefits.

Pomegranates

This fruit is also one that is packed full of antioxidants and anti-inflammatory components. It has even been suggested that it functions maximally in helping to prevent cancer; since it contains some anti-cancer properties. This is according to research published in the Journal of Advanced Biomedical Research in the year 2014.

Greek Yogurt

This is also another staple of the Mediterranean diet. Dairy components of the diet need to be consumed in moderate amounts. As a result, opting for Greek yogurt is ideal since it is a source of low or non-saturated fat food.

Arugula

The leafy green veggies such as the arugula are consumed in abundance in this diet. The meal plan entails eating green leafy vegetables more times than normal to reduce the risk of developing Alzheimer's disease.

Farro

As mentioned earlier, whole grains are an integral part of the Mediterranean diet. This delightful grain meal offers a satisfying source of protein and fiber. The consumption of whole grains is linked with a reduced risk of developing conditions such as heart disease, stroke, colorectal cancer, and type 2 diabetes.

Some other Mediterranean diet-compliant foods you can eat include, Broccoli, Chia seeds, Kale, Quinoa, Strawberries, Avocado, Blueberries, etc.

AVOID THESE FOODS WHEN ON THE DIET

Red meat

The Mediterranean diet as a whole is not big on red meat. And its consumption in large amounts is not advised. The meal plan has a vegetarian angle to it and it mostly makes use of animal protein as only a compliment and not as the main dish.

Refined sugars

Aside from refined sugars and all its attendant side effects, it is also not accepted as part of the Mediterranean diet. The meal plan does not require the use of lots of sugars, so instead, it is advised that a beginner or one starting on the diet should avoid sugar and anything that resembles it. This includes most baked foods and syrup-sweetened drinks like artificial juices and soda.

If you have a sweet tooth, it is advisable to turn to honey, fruits, or baked foods made with natural sweeteners like honey and cinnamon to get your fix.

Hard liquor

This must have been mentioned at one point or the other. As far as the Mediterranean diet is concerned, hard liquors such as tequila and Vodka are not allowed. If you are one that drinks alcohol on a consistent basis, you might need to stick to red wine as opposed to hard liquors.

It is advised that the freedom this diet gives to take at least a cup or at maximum two (2) cups of red wine does not mean the concerned individual should drink a whole bottle of wine with every meal. Moderation is advised.

GETTING STARTED WITH THE DIET

Effort

During the learning curve while getting used to the Mediterranean diet you may experience several issues. One thing you should become familiar with is the fact that it allows for experimentation and a lot of variety.

Take the time to plan your meals in advance. Shop for fresh produce at least twice a week. Take note to stock foods you can easily boil or grill like many Mediterranean diet foods out there. Keep the usual pantry staples such as canned tomatoes, whole grains, tuna, pasta, and olive oil.

Other things you should know

There are a few things you should also take note. One is that if you are looking for a long term, and productive way of achieving that change you have always wanted, the Mediterranean diet is really the way to go. With this new meal plan currently garnering attention the world over, you get to approach food and eating in a new way. You progressively learn how to consume food in moderation.

PRACTICAL DIET GUIDELINES:

✓ This cannot be overstated; as one of the first things to do is to start on a foundation of vegetables, whole grains, nuts, beans, and seeds. Whole grains make up the whole of the diet in the Mediterranean meal plan and snacking on them reduces the risk of developing cancer and heart disease. It is recommended that each meal should contain at least one serving of grains such as bread, pasta, or rice.

✓ Fruits and vegetables are the other staples of the diet that should not be ignored. They are key components. Their consumption has optimum health benefits as they're linked to lower risks of stroke or heart disease. As one targeting to be fully compliant to the dictates of the Mediterranean diet, one of the things to do is to at least aim for 2 servings of vegetables and fruits per meal.

✓ Legumes such as lentils and beans are also advised. They are an undeniable source of protein in the diet. So get familiar with them. Fish like salmon, tuna, and herring should be consumed at least twice a week. Red meat is also prohibited but if you are bent on eating it, do take note that its consumption should not be more than 3-4 Oz per week.

✓ As usual, moderate and constant physical activity is advised when on the Mediterranean diet. Try simple exercises like walking or gardening for about 30 minutes a day. Olive oil is also an excellent alternative to margarine and butter. And do you know that cooking tomatoes with olive oil go a long way in increasing the absorption of lycopene which is an antioxidant effective in fighting diseases.

The Mediterranean diet is super sustainable and fun to latch onto at the same time. So as for the many recipes, this meal plan has, if you are not digging into your well-prepared bowl of oatmeal, chopped apples, and walnuts, you are downing Greek yogurt with fresh almonds or berries. There are many cool ways of enjoying the Mediterranean diet.

MEDITERRANEAN BREAKFAST DIET RECIPES

The Breakfast Hash with Brussels Sprouts and Sweet Potatoes

Time: 40 minutes | Servings 1

Kcal 206, Carbs 19.3g/0.70oz, Protein 9.7g/0.34oz, Fat 11g/0.40oz, Fiber 4.8g/0.20oz

INGREDIENTS

- 1 medium-sized sweet potato, finely chopped
- 51g/3 cups of Brussels sprouts
- 1 healthy pinch of sea salt and black pepper
- 15ml/1 tablespoon of avocado oil
- 3 cloves of minced garlic
- 30ml/2 teaspoon of avocado oil
- 184g/¾ cup of finely diced Jonagold apple or diced Fuji
- ½ of a medium yellow, red, or white onion, chopped finely
- 34g/2 tablespoon of dried currants
- 17g/1 tablespoon of fresh minced sage
- 2 heaped cups of fresh spinach
- 4 large eggs
- 245g/1 cup of spicy pork sausage or chicken. Although as another option, you can buy local and organic meat if possible

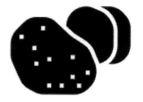

PREPARATION

1. As usual with all the methods of cooking out there, first preheat the oven to about 400 degrees and line the baking sheet with good quality parchment paper. After doing this, proceed to add Brussels and sweet potato to the baking sheet. Drizzle lightly with oil and then season with a dash of pepper and salt to taste.

2. Afterward, toss it all around to coat; bake for some minutes say about 25 minutes until it is golden brown or tender. Then make sure you toss it halfway point to allow for oven cooking. While in the meantime, you heat a moderately sized skillet over medium heat. Once it is hot, add the apple, garlic, currants, sage and then Sauté for about three minutes till they are slightly fragrant and golden brown while still stirring it occasionally.

3. Based on personal discretion, add veggie sausage or sausage and Sauté until it is golden brown, then cook through for some minutes. After this, you can use a spoon to break the sausage into small pieces.

4. After the sausage is properly cooked, add the spinach, cover, and cook for some minutes until it has wilted. Then stir in the roasted Brussels sprouts and sweet potato. Turn the heat off and set it aside for serving. Meanwhile, you should heat a separate skillet over moderate heat. Once it is hot, sprinkle a little oil and add the number of eggs you want, one egg per day is recommended.

5. To cook the egg, crack them in the pan and cook for some minutes, uncovered. Then proceed to cover with the lid in the last minutes so as to allow for the egg whites to cook while still keeping the yolk soft enough. As an alternative plan, you can choose to cook or scramble the eggs.

6. Lastly, enjoy the hash as it is, then you can decide to garnish with hot sauce or fresh herbs. Then the leftovers can be stored cool in the refrigerator for about 3-4 days or in the freezer for up to a month.

Shak Shuka with Tofu 'FETA'

Time: 40 minutes | Servings 1

Kcal 165, Carbs 14.4g/0.51oz, Protein 9g/0.32oz, Fat 9.2g/0.33oz, Fiber 3.8g/0.13oz

INGREDIENTS

- 245g/1 cup of diced white onion
- 2 cloves of garlic properly minced
- 15ml/1 tablespoon of olive oil
- A red bell pepper
- 2 (400g/14.5oz) cans of diced tomatoes
- 17g/1 teaspoon of smoked paprika
- 17g/1 teaspoon of Cumin
- 5 good quality eggs
- 4g/¼ teaspoon of salt and pepper to taste

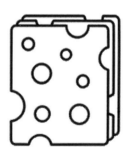

PREPARATION

1. As for the vegetables, preheat the oven to around 375F and then proceed to heat the oil in an oven-safe skillet over moderate heat. After, add garlic, onion, and bell pepper. Then cook until it has softened for about 5 minutes.

2. For the tomatoes add the canned tomatoes and then mash it with a fork till it forms a thick, chunky sauce. Allow the tomatoes to cook for some time, simmer till a thick sauce develops after about 10-15 minutes. Stir in the spices, the salt and pepper as usual to taste.

3. For the eggs, using the back of a spoon, form makeshift holes in the tomato sauce, then crack one egg into each hole. You can use as many eggs as you want. To bake, transfer the skillet to an oven that has earlier been preheated and cook uncovered for some minutes. Or until the egg whites are cooked.

4. You can then remove them when they are still a little soft on the insides and proceed to serve almost immediately with herbs, crumbled feta, or bread for dipping. In order to make it dairy-free, you can omit the feta cheese and instead make some tofu feta in its place. Spice it up by adding harissa paste, a moderate quantity, or make it more satisfying by adding chickpeas to the tomato sauce. Chickpeas, remember?

Mediterranean Diet Scrambled Eggs

Time: 20 minutes | Servings 1

Kcal 249, Carbs 17g/0.6oz, Proteins 13g/0.50oz, Fats 14g/0.50oz, Fiber 4g/0.14oz

INGREDIENTS

- 15ml/1 tablespoon of oil
- 2 sliced spring onions
- 8 quartered cherry tomatoes
- 4 eggs
- Black pepper
- 1g/¼ teaspoon of dried oregano
- 34g/2 tablespoon of sliced black olives
- 17g/1 tablespoon of capers
- 1 sliced yellow pepper and fresh parsley to serve

PREPARATION

1. As usual, heat the oil in a suitable frying pan, add diced pepper, and the chopped spring onions. Cook for some minutes over medium heat until they get soft. After this, add the tomatoes, capers, and olives, then cook for like a minute.

2. The eggs should be cracked into the pan and it should be scrambled immediately with a spoon or a spatula. Then proceed to add a lot of black pepper and oregano and stir until the eggs are fully cooked. Serve almost immediately and you can decide to top with fresh parsley if preferred.

Avocado Tomato Gouda Socca Pizza

Time: 50 minutes | Servings 2
Kcal 416, Carbs 36.6g/1.3oz, Protein15.4g/0.54oz, Fiber 9.6g/0.34oz, Fat 24.5g/0.9oz

INGREDIENTS

- 1g/¼ teaspoon of pepper and sea salt
- 30ml/2 tablespoon of avocado or olive oil
- 4g/1 teaspoon of minced garlic (2 cloves)

- 375ml/1¼ cup of cold water
- 4g/1teaspoon of onion powder or any preferable herbal-based seasoning of choice
- 150g/1¼ cup g of garbanzo/chickpea bean flour

Socca Pizza Toppings:

- ½ avocado
- 1 Roma Sliced
- Red pepper flakes
- 1 Roma Tomato Sliced
- 56g/2oz Gouda, properly sliced thin. Sometimes Goat milk works well in preparing Gouda too
- 32g/¼ cup of tomato sauce
- Sprouted green vegetables such as kale, broccoli, and onion greens
- Salt and Pepper to sprinkle on the top after preparing, also add to taste

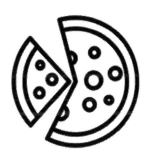

PREPARATION

1. When it comes to preparing this absolute delight, the first thing to do is to first mix the flour, make use of 2 tablespoons of olive oil, herbs, and water together. Mix very well until you have a consistent mixture and then allow the mixture to sit for about 15-20 minutes at room temperature.

2. While you have left the mixture you have sitting, preheat the oven to boil, and then place the oven to heat for some minutes. And while the oven is preheating, slice your vegetables cleanly and also set it aside. After using the oven mitts, remove the pan after 10 minutes. Add one tablespoon of oil to the pan and swirl it around so it coats the pan.

3. When all this is done, pour in the batter you have made and tilt the pan slightly till the batter fills the whole of the pan. After doing this, reduce the heat on the oven and place it back for about 10 minutes and until it is set. Do note that if the pan is a big one, the resulting pizza will be thinner and it will bake faster in no time.

4. Proceed to remove from the oven. This should allow you to slide the pizza onto a heat-safe surface or a stone. After this, add a bunch of microgreens or sprouts on the top with any additional toppings you prefer. Salt, pepper, onions, red pepper fits into this category.

5. After following these steps to the letter, sprinkle olive oil on the top, slice, and serve.

Greek Omelet Casserole

Time: 33 minutes | Servings 1

Kcal 186, Carbs 5g/0.17oz, Protein 10g/0.35oz, Fat 13g/0.50oz, Fiber 3g/0.11oz

INGREDIENTS

- 500ml/2 cups of whole milk
- 2 healthy cloves of garlic, properly minced
- 12 eggs, yes such a number. It is an omelet casserole after all
- 140g/5oz of fully sundried tomatoes, and feta dried cheese, crumbled
- 230g/8oz of fresh spinach
- 340g/12oz of artichoke salad
- 4g/1 teaspoon of salt
- 4g/1 teaspoon of lemon pepper, and dried oregano
- 60ml/4 teaspoons of olive oil, divided

PREPARATION

1. As usual, preheat the oven to around 375 degrees F and the move to chop the artichoke salad and fresh herbs. After this, set a suitable skillet over medium heat and add a tablespoon of olive oil. After this, sauté the garlic and spinach on medium heat for about three (3) minutes until it is wilted.

2. Proceed to oil a moderately-sized baking dish, layer the artichoke salad, and spinach in the dish. Then in a medium bowl, whisk the eggs, herbs, milk, salt, lemon, and pepper. Pour the mixture over the vegetables while also sprinkling with feta cheese. Bake in the center of the oven for about half an hour until it is firm in the center.

Cauliflower Fritters with Hummus

Time: 35 minutes | Servings 2
Kcal 480, Carbs 59g/2.10z, Fiber 10g/0.35oz, Fats 16g/0.56oz, Protein 18g/0.63oz

INGREDIENTS

- 50ml/2 ½ tablespoons of olive oil, divided and some more for frying
- 2 (430g/15oz) cans chickpeas fully divided
- 2g/½ teaspoon of salt
- Hummus, depending on choice for topping
- Diced Green onion, for Garnish
- 128g/1 cup onion, finely chopped, and about half a small onion
- 250g/2 cups of cauliflower, cut into small pieces with about ½ a large head
- 34g/2 tablespoons of garlic, properly minced

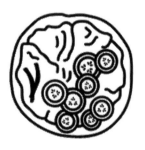

PREPARATION

1. As usual, preheat the oven to around 400 F, then rinse and drain a can of the chickpeas then place them on a paper towel so you can dry them very well. Afterward, place the peas in a properly sized bowl, removing any of the loose skins that come off. Proceed to scrape them out into a pan, make sure you do not overcrowd them on the pan, and then sprinkle with salt and pepper to taste.

2. Proceed to bake the chickpeas for like 20 minutes, stir them, and further bake for some more minutes until they are very crispy. After this, transfer the peas to a capable food processor and process them until they have finally been broken down. Do not turn them into flour as it is ideal if you still leave some for texture. Place the result in a bowl and still set aside.

3. Heat the olive oil remaining in a large pan on medium heat. Add the garlic and onion and cook until it is lightly golden brown, add the cauliflower and cook for some more minutes till it also turns golden. Cook the cauliflower until it is fork-tender, and the onions are caramelized and golden brown while stirring often. A task that takes about 5 minutes' maximum.

4. Transfer the cauliflower mixture you have to the food processor, drain and rinse the remaining can of chickpeas, add into the processor, together with a reasonable pinch of pepper and salt to taste. Move to blend all together till it is smooth and the mixture starts to turn into a ball and then stop to scrape down the sides until it is necessary.

5. Turn the cauliflower mixture in a large bowl, then add half a cup of roasted chickpea crumbs. You do not have to use all the crumbs. After this, stir very well and combine very easily. Then pour enough oil to cover the surface of the large pan and then heat on medium heat. After this, cook the patties until they are golden brown for a few minutes, flip and cool again. Work in small batches. When you are done, serve with green onions and devour almost immediately.

Greek Salad Sushi

Time: 15 minutes | Servings 3

Kcal 54, Carbs 5.2g/0.18oz, Protein 4g/0.142oz, Fat 1.5g/0.05oz, Fiber 0.6g/0.02oz

INGREDIENTS

- 125g/½ a cup of Greek yogurt
- 1 good quality cucumber
- 1 clove of minced garlic
- 10ml/2 teaspoons of lemon juice, about 10ml
- Salt and pepper to taste
- 30g/¼ cup of crumbled feta cheese
- 61g/¼ cup of diced onion
- A teaspoon of fresh dill
- Bell pepper sliced into half

PREPARATION

1. The first thing to do is to chop off the ends of the cucumber, and also making use of a vegetable peeler or mandolin to peel thin slices all along, in a lengthwise manner. After this, set the cut slices on paper towels and cover. Allow it to dry, while you make the tzatziki.

2. It is simple to make the TzaTziki, all you have to do is combine all the other ingredients which include lemon, garlic, salt, pepper, dill, and yogurt.

3. After doing this, the next step is to spread the tzatziki on a slice of a cucumber and then top with feta, onion, and pepper. Roll it up and secure with a toothpick and then continue in the same manner till you have exhausted all the ingredients.

Muesli with Raspberries

Time: 5 minutes | Servings 1
Kcal 287, Carbs 51.8g/1.83oz, Protein 13g/0.5oz, Fiber 13.3g/0.46oz

INGREDIENTS

- 245g/1 cup of raspberries
- About 74g/⅓ cup of muesli, and some low-fat milk

PREPARATION

1. All you need to do is top the muesli with raspberries and serve with milk generously. In all, we are combining 2 starch, a fruit, and ½ cup of low-fat milk.

Banana Split Yogurt

Time: 5 minutes | Servings 2

Kcal 281, Carbs 2g/0.07oz, Fats 29g/1oz, Protein 4g/0.14oz, Fiber 4g/0.14oz

INGREDIENTS

- 🍽 250ml/1 cup of Greek yogurt
- 🍽 ½ sliced banana
- 🍽 10ml/2 teaspoons of jam
- 🍽 8g/2 teaspoons of cacao nibs

PREPARATION

1. Combine all the ingredients in a single bowl and serve!

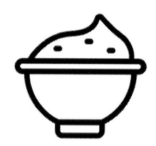

Quick and Easy Greek Salad

Time: 10 minutes | Servings 1

Kcal 390, Carbs 53.8g/1.89oz, Proteins 19.1g/0.67oz, Fats 11.5g/0.4oz, Fiber 10.8g/0.38oz

INGREDIENTS

- 1 full tomato
- ¼ red onion
- 3 black olives
- ¼ yellow pepper
- 50g/1.76oz salad leaves
- 30g/1.05oz feta cheese
- 1 bagel
- 17g/1 tablespoon fat free vinaigrette

PREPARATION

1. Begin by chopping the pepper, onions, olives and tomatoes.
2. Combine the chopped veggies with the salad leaves and top with the dressing.
3. Now put in the diced Feta cheese.
4. Finally toast the bagel before serving.

MEDITERRANEAN DIET LUNCH RECIPES

The Classic Mediterranean Salad

Time: 5 minutes | Servings 4
Kcal 132, Carbs 2g/0.07oz, Protein 2g/0.07oz, Fat 12g/0.42oz, Fiber 2g/0.07oz

INGREDIENTS

- 30ml/2 tablespoons of red wine vinegar
- 2g/½ teaspoon of minced fresh garlic

- A pinch of salt and black pepper
- 74g/⅓ cup of good quality, virgin olive oil
- ½ teaspoon of Italian seasoning

For the salad:

- 128g/1 cup of cherry or grape tomatoes
- ½ finely sliced red onions
- 32g/¼ cup of crumbled feta cheese
- 480g/2½ cups of packed salad greens, preferably spinach

- A small can of sliced black olives properly drained
- 245g/2 cups of thinly sliced cucumbers, cut into the half-moon shape

PREPARATION

1. In a moderately-sized bowl, whisk all the dressing together and set it all aside. After, in another bowl put together all the salad and drizzle lightly with the dressing to evenly coat the greens in the bowl with enough dressing. Your salad is ready; and you may need to also refrigerate.

Mediterranean Veggie Sandwich

Time: 5 minutes | Servings 2

Kcal 112, Carbs 14.4g/0.51oz, Protein 2g/0.07oz, Fiber 13.3g/0.46oz, Fat 9.2g/0.33oz

INGREDIENTS

- 1 whole leaf of fresh lettuce
- 32g/¼ cup of sprouts
- 2 slices of good quality wheat bread
- 51g/3 tablespoons of cilantro jalapeno hummus
- 34g/2 tablespoons of crumbled feta cheese
- 2 whole peppadew peppers, chopped
- 2 whole thin slices of cucumber
- 2 whole thin slices of tomato

PREPARATION

1. You can toast the bread if you wish, spread both slices of bread with hummus, and then layer on tomato, lettuce, red onions, cucumber, cheese, feta, and peppadew peppers. You can then slice the sandwich in half and serve almost immediately.

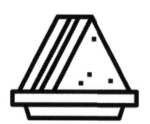

Falafel Kale Salad with the Best Tahini Dressing

Time: 10 minutes | Servings 3
Kcal 499, Fat 31.1g/1.09oz, Protein 15.7g/0.5oz, Carbs 44.8g/1.6oz, Fiber 13.2g/0.46oz

INGREDIENTS

- 430g/15oz can of white beans, rinsed and drained
- 2 slices of pita bread cut into squares
- 1 Jalapeno chopped finely
- ½ of the red onion sliced thinly
- 500g/4 cups kale cut in bite pieces
- 1-2 juiced lemons
- A recipe of simple crispy vegan falafel balls
- A recipe for the best Tahini dressing too is also needed

PREPARATION

1. Making the falafel salad is very easy, all you need to do is to place the kale in a bowl and drizzle on it with lemon juice. Depending on the quantity of your kale and how juicy the lemons are. But to take note you massage the kale for some seconds so the lemon juice is incorporated into it. Place in the fridge until it is ready to use.

2. Prepare the tahini dressing according to the earlier laid out instructions and also place in the fridge till it is ready for use, also prepare the simple crispy vegan falafel according to instructions. A random search on the internet would show this.

3. Then move to assemble the salads, divide the kale between the bowls and then top each with three (3) falafel balls, the white beans, the red onion, the Jalapeno, and Pita slices. Finally, proceed to drizzle the dressing over each bowl you make, serve, and enjoy almost immediately.

Mediterranean Quinoa Bowls with Roasted Red Pepper Sauce

Time: 15 minutes | Servings 4
Kcal 349, Carbs 30.9g/1.08oz, Fiber 6g/0.2oz, Protein 10.9g/0.40oz, Fat 25.6g/0.9oz

INGREDIENTS

- Enough juice of just 1 lemon
- 125ml/½ cup of olive oil
- 60g/½ of almonds
- 2g/½ teaspoon of salt
- A clove of garlic
- 1 (450g/16oz) jar roasted with enough red pepper, and properly drained
- 60g/½ cup of almond
- Feta cheese
- Kalamata olives
- Thinly sliced red onion
- Hummus
- Spinach, cucumber, or kale. It is said that for the Mediterranean bowls, you can build up your own bowls based on what you like
- Fresh basil or parsley

PREPARATION

1. All the sauce should first be placed in a suitable food processor; a blender is also common in some areas. Process or blend until it is smooth; as the texture must be textured and thick.

2. Cook the quinoa according to the instructions on its package. When it is done, build a Mediterranean quinoa bowl. You can decide to store the leftovers in separate containers and then assemble each bowl just before serving. Most especially the greens and sauces as it will get soggy when stored with all the other. Do note that for the vegan version, replace the feta cheese with white beans.

Lemon and Parmesan Chicken with Zucchini Noodles

Time: 20 minutes | Servings 2
Kcal 1298, Carbs 62g/2.2oz, Fat 65g/2.3oz, Protein 131g/5oz, Fiber 20g/0.71oz

INGREDIENTS

- 4g/1 teaspoon of fine sea salt
- 2 packages of green giant veggie spirals
- 10ml/2 teaspoons of oil
- 4 garlic cloves, minced
- 34g/2 tablespoons of high-quality butter
- Lemon slices, for garnish
- Parsley for garnish
- 680g/1½lb of boneless skinless chicken breast, cut into bite-sized pieces
- 147g/⅔ cup of broth
- 74g/⅓ cup of parmesan
- 34g/2 tablespoons of dried oregano

PREPARATION

1. One of the first things to do is to cook the Zucchini noodles according to the instructions on the package. Do make sure you drain it very well. After this, heat the oil in a large skillet over medium heat, season the chicken with enough pepper and salt, and the brown chicken pieces. Do this for about 3 or 4 minutes per side of the chicken, depending on how thick the chicken is. You can cook in batches. Remove the chicken from the pan.

2. Also to the skillet, add the garlic you have and cook until it becomes fragrant. Allow it to rest for some seconds. Add the oregano, lemon zest, and butter, pour in the chicken broth to deglaze while making sure that all the browned bits on the bottom of the pan. You can turn up the heat to medium-high to bring the chicken and the sauce to boil. Lower the heat and stir it in the parmesan cheese.

3. Place the chicken back in the pan and simmer gently for some minute until the sauce has reduced and its thickness has increased. Taste and adjust the seasoning as appropriate. This you can serve warm over the Zucchini noodles and then garnish generously with lemon slices and parsley.

The Lemony Orzo Salad

Time: 5 minutes: Servings 3

INGREDIENTS

- 245g/1 cup of roughly chopped fresh basil leaves
- 245g/1 cup of roughly chopped fresh mint
- 60ml/¼ cup of olive oil
- Sea salt and freshly cracked black pepper for seasoning
- As options, you can make use of crumbled goat or feta cheese

- 1 diced, English cucumber
- 340g/12oz of uncooked orzo or any suitable pasta shape
- Two handfuls of chopped fresh baby spinach
- A can of chickpeas, rinsed and drained
- 2 lemons zested and juiced

PREPARATION

1. First cook the pasta in a large, suitable stockpot. Do take note to pre-salt the water until al dente according to the instructions on the package. Drain the pasta accordingly and then rinse thoroughly in a strainer with cold water until the pasta is chilled. Move to transfer the pasta to a large mixing bowl.

2. After this, add the remaining to the mixing bowl, toss until it is evenly combined. Then taste, season with pinches of pepper and salt to taste as mentioned. You can also add enough lemon juice if you like.

3. Your salad is done. Serve almost immediately and it can be refrigerated for up to 3 days.

Couscous and Chickpea Salad

Time: 5 minutes | Servings 2
Kcal 481, Carbs 67.6g/2.4oz, Fat 16.7g/0.60oz, Protein 17.3g/0.61oz, Fiber 13.4g/0.50oz

INGREDIENTS

- 68g/4 tablespoons of basil vinaigrette, you can check for the associated recipe for it
- 128g/1 cup of finely chopped kale
- 85g/⅔ of rinsed canned chickpeas
- 96g/¾ cup of cooked whole meat couscous

PREPARATION

1. This is also very simple, all you need to do is to combine chickpeas, the dressing, kale, couscous in a medium-sized bowl. After this, you can serve immediately or decide to refrigerate in a sealable container for about 4 days. In case you want to make it ahead, you can make it, cover, and refrigerate for up to 4 days.

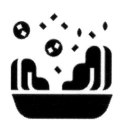

Beet and Winter Shrimp Salad

Time: 5 minutes | Servings 2
Kcal 171, Fat 7.7g/0.30oz, Carbs 16.3g/0.57oz, Proteins 4.3g/0.20oz, Fibers 4.0g/0.14oz

INGREDIENTS

- 245g/1 cup of lightly packed watercress
- 245g/1 cup of cooked beet wedges
- 122g/½ cup of already made zucchini noodles
- 490g/2 of lightly packed arugula

- 122g/½ cup of thinly sliced fennel
- 122g/½ cup of cooked barley
- Fennel fronds for the garnish
- 115g/4oz of cooked, peeled shrimp, the tails left on if desired

For the vinaigrette:

- Make use of 15ml/1tablespoon of red or white wine vinegar
- 2g/½ a teaspoon of Dijon Mustard
- 2g/½a teaspoon of minced shallot

- 2g/½ teaspoon of ground pepper
- A pinch of salt
- 30ml/2 tablespoons of extra-virgin olive oil

PREPARATION

1. Arrange the greens, watercress, beets, fennel, barley, shrimp, and zucchini on a very large dinner plate. After this, whisk the oil, mustard, shallot, pepper and salt, vinegar in a small bowl. Drizzle over the salad, garnish generously with fennel fronds if you like, and your salad is ready.

Greek Zucchini and Walnut Salad

Time: 20 minutes | Servings 2
Kcal 595, Carbs 8g/0.28oz, Fats 58g/2.05oz, Protein 9g/0.32oz, Fiber 7g/0.24oz

INGREDIENTS

- 🍽 32g/¼ cup of freshly cut chives
- 🍽 15ml/1 tablespoon of olive oil
- 🍽 2 zucchini
- 🍽 1 finely minced clove of garlic
- 🍽 10ml/2 teaspoons lemon juice
- 🍽 190ml/¾ cup of vegan mayonnaise
- 🍽 30ml/2 tablespoons of olive oil
- 🍽 2g/½ teaspoon of salt
- 🍽 1g/¼ teaspoon of chili powder
- 🍽 A head of romaine lettuce
- 🍽 100g/3½ cup of chopped walnuts
- 🍽 115g/4oz of arugula lettuce
- 🍽 Pepper and salt

PREPARATION

1. Combine and whisk all the ingredients for making the dressing. Once mixed thoroughly, set aside to develop and blend flavors.
2. Put the romaine lettuce, chives, and arugula in a single bowl.
3. Cut and split the zucchini along the length then remove the seeds. Further cut the zucchini across into half-inch slices.
4. On a pan, bring olive oil to heat before adding the chopped zucchini. Add some pepper and a pinch of salt to your liking.
5. Sauté till you achieve a light brown color.
6. Combine the salad and zucchini before mixing thoroughly.
7. Roast nuts in the same pan. Add some pepper and salt to taste.
8. Serve the nuts on the salad and top with the salad dressing.

The Mediterranean Vegan Salad

Time: 15 minutes | Servings 4

Kcal 195, Carbs 10.9g/0.38oz, Proteins 2g/0.07oz, Fats 17.1g/0.6oz, Fiber 5.5g/0.19oz

INGREDIENTS

- 3 large tomatoes
- Pepper and salt
- 32g/¼ cup of baby tomatoes
- Juice from ½ a lemon
- 1 avocado
- 30ml/2 tablespoons of balsamic vinegar
- 1 Persian cucumber
- 30ml/2 tablespoons olive oil
- ½ red onion
- 2g/½ teaspoon of Dijon mustard
- Fresh basil

PREPARATION

1. Roughly cut the cucumber, onions, avocados, and tomatoes then put them on a serving dish.
2. Slice the baby tomatoes into halves and lay add to the dish.
3. Sprinkle chopped basil over the salad.
4. In a separate bowl, combine and whisk balsamic vinegar, olive oil, mustard, lemon juice pepper, and salt.
5. Empty the dressing atop the salad and serve.

MEDITERRANEAN DIET DINNER RECIPES

Slow-Cooker Mediterranean Stew

Time: 6 hours 30 minutes | Servings 2

Kcal 130, Carbs 30.5g/1.08oz, Proteins 3.4g/0.12oz, Fats 0.5g/0.02oz, Fiber 7.8g/0.28oz

INGREDIENTS

- 735g/3 cups of vegetable broth low in sodium
- 245g/1 cup of medium-sized onions chopped coarsely
- 4 cloves of garlic, properly minced
- 4g/1 teaspoon of dried oregano
- 2g/½ teaspoon of crushed red pepper
- 15ml/1 tablespoon of lemon juice
- 45ml/3 tablespoon of extra virgin olive oil
- Fresh basil leaves
- A bunch of Lacinato kale, chopped and stemmed. About eight (8) cups of them
- A can of no-salt included rinsed, and divided chickpeas
- 2 cans of no-salt-added fire-roasted tomatoes
- ¾ chopped carrot

- 6 lemon wedges

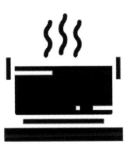

PREPARATION

1. This is very simple to prepare. First, you combine the tomatoes, onion, broth, garlic, carrot, oregano, crushed red pepper, and salt to taste in a 4-quart slow-cooking pot. Then cover and cook on low heat for about 6 hours.

2. After doing that, measure a quarter cup of the cooking liquid from the slow cooking pot into a small bowl, then add the chickpeas and mash with a fork until it appears smooth. Then add the mashed mix you have to the remaining in the slow cooker. Stir it in and combine; after, cover and cook till it is tender for about 30 minutes.

3. Lastly, ladle the stew into about six (6) bowls and then drizzle with oil, based on personal discretion nevertheless, after garnish with enough basil and then serve preferably with lemon wedges.

Greek Stuffed Mushroom Portobellos

Time: 25 minutes | Servings 4
Kcal 151, Carbs 6.6g/0.3oz, Protein 4.5g/0.16oz, Fat 8.5g/0.3oz, Fiber 1.8g/0.06oz

INGREDIENTS

- A clove of garlic minced
- 2g/½ teaspoon of ground pepper, divided
- 1g/¼ teaspoon of salt
- 45ml/3 tablespoons of extra virgin olive oil
- 4 good quality Portobello mushrooms wiped very clean with gills and stem removed
- 245g/1 cup of chopped spinach
- 122g/½ cup of quartered cherry tomatoes
- 122g/½ cup of crumbled cheese
- 34g/2 tablespoons of pitted and sliced Kalamata olives
- 17g/1 tablespoon of chopped fresh oregano

PREPARATION

1. Preheat the oven to a considerable extent, then move to combine the oil, pepper, garlic, and salt in a suitable bow. Afterward, making use of an appropriate silicone brush coat the mushrooms with the oil mixture and then place the mushrooms on the already rimmed baking sheet until it is soft.

2. In the meantime, combine the tomatoes, spinach, olives, feta, oregano, and the remaining oil in a medium-sized bowl and after the mushrooms have softened, remove them from the ovens and fill them with the spinach mixture you have and then bake until the tomatoes have wilted. Just for about 10 minutes. Serve almost immediately.

Mediterranean Ravioli with Artichokes and Olives

Time: 15 minutes | Servings 4
Kcal 454, Fat 19.2g/0.7oz, Carbs 60.1g/2.12oz, Fiber 13.1g/0.46oz, Protein 15g/0.53oz

INGREDIENTS

- 122g/½ cup of oil-packed sun-dried tomatoes, and well-drained
- A package of frozen quartered artichoke hearts thawed
- 2 (230g/8oz) frozen packages of ricotta ravioli
- 28g/1oz can of no salt added rinsed cannellini beans
- 62g/¼ cup of Kalamata sliced olives
- 51g/3 tablespoons of roasted pine nuts
- 62g/¼ cup of chopped fresh basil

PREPARATION

1. Boil water in a large pot and then cook the ravioli according to the directions. Afterward drains and toss it with a tablespoon of oil that has been set aside. Then move to heat the remaining tablespoon of oil in a non-stick skillet all over medium heat. Add the beans and artichokes and beans, sauté until it is heated through and through for about 3 minutes.

2. The last thing to do is to fold in the ravioli you have cooked, the sun-dried tomatoes, pine nuts, basil, and olives. Serve almost immediately.

Prosciutto Pizza with Corn and Arugula

Time: 20 minutes | Servings 4
Kcal 436, Fat 19.9g/0.70oz, Carbs 53.1g/1.87oz, Protein 18.3g/0.65oz, Fiber 3g/0.11oz

INGREDIENTS

- 450g/1lb of pizza, preferably whole-wheat pizza
- A clove of garlic, preferably minced
- 245g/1 cup of part-skim shredded mozzarella cheese
- 28g/1oz of thinly sliced prosciutto, torn into one-inch pieces
- 367g/1½ cups of arugula
- 122g/½ cup of torn, fresh basil
- 1g/¼ teaspoon of ground pepper
- Fresh corn kennels

PREPARATION

1. The first thing to do as usual is to grill most preferably under medium heat. Roll out a reasonable amount of dough on an already floured surface, beat it into a 12-inch oval, and transfer to a similarly floured baking sheet. Combine it with one tablespoon of oil and garlic in a small bowl, bring the garlic, oil, cheese, corn, prosciutto, and the dough to the grill.

2. Oil the grill rack properly and transfer the crust to the grill. Take time to grill the dough as much as possible, until it is lightly browned and puffed. This should take just a few minutes. After this, flip over the crust and spread the oil from garlic on it. top it generously with corn, cheese, and prosciutto.

3. Grill the combination, while it is covered with the cheese till it is melted and the crust is browned some more. Do this for some minutes and then return the pizza to the baking sheet. Top the pizza with arugula, pepper, and basil. Then drizzle the remaining with a tablespoon of oil and serve.

Greek Burgers with Herb-Feta Sauce

Time: 25 minutes | Servings 4
Kcal 375, Fat 18.1g/0.64oz, Carbs 23.5g/0.83oz, Protein 29.8g/1.05oz, Fiber 2.5g/0.088oz

INGREDIENTS

- 10ml/2 teaspoons of lemon juice
- Small red onion
- 450g/1lb lamb or ground beef
- 245g/1 cup of sliced cucumber
- Plum, sliced tomato
- 2 whole-wheat pitas, split, halved and warmed
- 245g/1 cup of fat-free plain Greek yogurt
- 72g/¼ cup of crumbled feta cheese
- 51g/3 tablespoons of chopped fresh oregano, divided

PREPARATION

1. Preheat the grill to medium-high or preheat broiler or preheat the broiler to high. After this, mix the feta, a tablespoon of oregano, lemon zest, lemon juice, and a teaspoon of salt in a small bowl. Then cut about ¼ inches of thick slices of onion to make about a quarter of the cup.

2. After this, mix the meat and chopped onions and meat in a bowl and with the remaining two 2) tablespoons of oregano and a half teaspoon each of salt and pepper to taste. Then move away from each of the four (4) patties which will be about 3 by 4 inches each.

3. Then grill or broil the burgers as you please, then turn once, while still making use of an instant thermometer to regulate the temperature. Serve in pita halves, then with onion slices, cucumber, tomato, and sauce to taste.

Salmon Pita Sandwich

Time: 5 minutes | Servings 2
Kcal 239, Fats 7.1g/0.25oz, Carbs 19g/0.67oz, Protein 24.8g/0.87oz, Fiber 2.3g/0.081oz

INGREDIENTS

- 🍽 8g/2 teaspoons of fresh dill chopped
- 🍽 2g/½ teaspoon of prepared horseradish
- 🍽 30ml/2 tablespoons of plain non-fat yogurt
- 🍽 125ml/½ cup of watercress
- 🍽 ½ a 6-inch whole-wheat pita bread
- 🍽 85g/3oz of flaked canned sockeye salmon
- 🍽 10ml/2 teaspoons of lemon juice

PREPARATION

1. The directions for preparing this delicacy are so simple and all you need to do is to combine the lemon juice, horseradish, dill, yogurt, in a small bowl. After combining, stir in the salmon. Then stuff the pita with half the watercress and salmon salad.

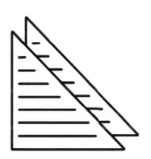

Gluten-Free Pasta Mediterranean Style

Time: 5 minutes | Servings 2
Kcal 165, Carbs 14.4g/0.51oz, Protein 9g/0.32oz, Fat 9.2g/0.33oz, Fiber 3.8g/0.13oz

INGREDIENTS

- Avocados for a start
- A pinch of black pepper
- 1g/¼ teaspoon of ground cumin
- The same amount of red pepper flakes too
- A pint of cherry tomatoes
- 2 medium-sized Chinese eggplants which are diced into small cubes

- 4g/1 teaspoon of salt
- A great package of brown rice spaghetti, cooked according to all the pre-written instructions and cooled
- 17g/1 tablespoon each of finely chopped mint, parsley, cilantro, and Dill

For the Lemon Dressing:

- 1g/¼ teaspoon of granulated sugar
- 125ml/½ cup of olive oil, and 4g/1 teaspoon Dijon mustard
- Pinch of black pepper
- 4 large cloves of garlic, pressed through a garlic press
- 1 Zest of lemon
- 1g/¼ teaspoon of salt and lemon juice

PREPARATION

1. First, preheat the oven to around 400 and then line the baking sheet with parchment paper. After, making use of a large bowl, toss the diced eggplant and the cherry tomatoes. Add about 3-4 tablespoons of oil, the salt, pepper, red pepper flakes, cumin, granulated garlic come onto the already lined baking sheet until golden and it is tender.

2. Make sure you have a cooked and cooled brown rice pasta ready in a large bowl. Add some of the lemon dressing and the cherry tomatoes, egg-plant mixture. Sprinkle in the chopped herbs and add everything together gently. You might need to add some salt and pepper to taste. After this, serve immediately or keep chilled in a fridge.

3. For the Lemon dressing, all you have to do is to place all the ingredients a moderately sized bowl, seal the top and shake very well to allow the ingredients to properly emulsify. Make use of it immediately or you can choose to keep it cool in the fridge, this is for the lemon dressing.

Mediterranean Stuffed Sweet Potatoes with Chickpeas and Avocado Tahini

Time: 60 minutes | Servings 3

Kcal 127, Carbohydrates 38g/1.34oz, Fiber 8g/0.3oz, Protein 7g/0.25oz, Fat 2g/0.071oz

INGREDIENTS

- 8 medium-sized, good quality sweet potatoes and rinsed well
- For the marinated Chickpeas, make use of ½ red pepper, diced
- 15ml/1 tablespoon of fresh lemon juice
- ½ of red pepper, properly diced

- 45ml/3 tablespoons of extra virgin olive oil
- 15ml/1 tablespoon of lemon zest
- 17g/1 tablespoon of freshly chopped parsley
- 1g/¼ teaspoon of sea salt
- 1 (430g/15oz) can of chickpeas, rinsed and drained

For the Avocado Tahini Sauce:

- 60ml/¼ cup of water
- 61g/¼ cup of tahini
- 1medium-sized, ripe avocado
- 17g/1 tablespoon of fresh parsley
- 15ml/1 tablespoon of fresh lemon juice
- 1 clove of crushed garlic

PREPARATION

1. Preheat the oven to about 400F, and use a fork to pierce a few holes in the sweet potatoes you have down, to allow the air to escape. Afterward, place them all on the baking sheet and proceed to bake for some minutes or even up to an hour till it is tender to touch. Note that the larger the potatoes, the more time it takes to bake.

2. Meanwhile, when the potatoes are being baked, start working on the chickpeas. In a moderately sized bowl, mix the chickpeas and the other required for marinating. Afterward, toss the chickpeas and marinate properly until they are well coated in the marinade.

3. Also to make the tahini sauce, add all the needed to make the sauce into a blender and blend till it is smooth. Add enough water, depending on the type of consistency you want. once you have a sauce smooth enough, transfer to a bowl and set aside.

4. For the assembly of all you have prepared, take the potatoes as tender as they are, set it aside, and allow it to cool. Cut down the middle of each potato, and taking enough care, spoon the chickpeas inside. Then top with the avocado tahini and also sprinkle the Papitas over the top coupled with crumbled up feta. They are best served fresh and you can also keep them for up to 2 days.

Casserole Fish with Mushroom and French Mustard

Time: 45 minutes | Servings 6

Kcal 858, Carbs 9g/0.32oz, Fats 74g/2.6oz, Proteins 39g/1.38oz, Fiber 4g/0.14oz

INGREDIENTS

- 4g/1 teaspoon of salt
- Pepper
- 34g/2 tablespoon of fresh parsley
- 34g/2 tablespoon of Dijon mustard
- 226g/8oz of shredded cheese
- 453g/1lb of mushrooms
- 100g/3½oz of butter
- 100g/3½oz of butter or olive oil
- 680g/1½lb of cod
- 680g/1½lb of cauliflower or broccoli

PREPARATION

1. Bring the oven to a temperature of 175°C/350°F.
2. Chop the mushrooms into wedges and fry in butter for 5 minutes until nice and soft before adding salt, parsley, and pepper to taste.
3. Introduce the whipping cream and mustard at a lower temperature and simmer for 5 minutes to achieve a thick sauce consistency.
4. Season the fish with salt and pepper. Spread some cheese over and top with the mushroom sauce then finish off the remaining cheese on top.
5. If the fish is frozen, let it cook for 30 minutes, otherwise, 25 minutes will be fine. Using a fork check if the fish is ready. You will know if the fish is cooked if it flakes easily on the fork.
6. Slice the broccoli or cauliflower into florets and parboil in salted water before straining and adding some oil or butter.
7. Mash, season with some salt and pepper then serve with the fish.

Roasted Vegetable Mediterranean

Time: 45 minutes | Servings 1

Kcal 854, Carbs 20.8g/0.73oz, Proteins 5.4g/0.19oz, Fats 87.1g/3.07oz, Fiber 5.2g/0.17oz

INGREDIENTS

- 🍽 250ml/1 cup of kale cut into ribbons
- 🍽 A pinch of crushed red pepper flakes
- 🍽 60ml/¼ cup of marinated artichoke hearts
- 🍽 Freshly ground black pepper and sea salt
- 🍽 60ml/¼ cup of Kalamata olives
- 🍽 17g/1 tablespoon of fresh parsley
- 🍽 32g/¼ cup of chopped walnuts
- 🍽 17g/1 tablespoon of nutritional yeast
- 🍽 34g/2 tablespoons of chopped sun dried tomatoes
- 🍽 15ml/1 tablespoon of olive oil
- 🍽 15ml/1 tablespoon of fresh lemon juice
- 🍽 ½ spaghetti squash with seeds removed

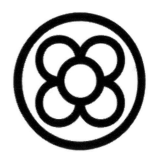

PREPARATION

1. Bring the oven to a temperature of 400°F before lining the baking sheet with parchment paper.

2. On one half of the baking sheet, place the squashes then top with some olive oil, pepper, and some sea salt.

3. Cook in the oven for 45 minutes having the cut side down.

4. Using a fork, scrap the stands far from the shell before adding some more salt to taste.

5. Now place the artichokes, tomatoes, walnuts, Kalamata olives, and kale atop the squashes.

6. Finally, drizzle with the lemon juice, some olive oil, and top with the freshly chopped parsley.

7. Add some red pepper if you so wish and enjoy!

28-Day Mediterranean Diet Meal Planner

To get the best out of the diet, here are some great ideas on how you can start planning your menu to derive premium benefits from the meal plan. With the Mediterranean diet, we would be giving you some ideas on the foods to prepare, with regards to your breakfast, lunch, and dinner.

DAY 1

Breakfast: The Caprese Avocado Toast
Time: 5 minutes | Servings 2
Kcal 338, Carbs, 25.8g/0.91oz, Proteins 12.8g/0.45oz, Fats 20.4g/0.72oz, Fiber 9.2g/0.32oz

INGREDIENTS

- 1 medium avocado, well halved and its pit removed
- 2 slices of a hearty sandwich bread such as the whole wheat bread, sourdough, etc.
- 8 grape tomatoes, halved
- 4 large fresh and good quality ciliegine, or bite-sized mozzarella balls, about 12 of them
- 34g/2 tablespoons of balsamic glaze

PREPARATION

1. It is very simple to prepare, just toast the bread and while it is toasting, proceed to mash all the avocados in a small bowl. After doing this, spread the mashed avocado over all the toast and then top each of the slices you have with basil leaves, tomatoes, mozzarella, and finally drizzle on top with balsamic glaze.
2. Serve immediately.

Lunch: The Classic Mediterranean Salad (See page 39)
Dinner: Slow-Cooker Mediterranean Stew (See page 51)

DAY 2

Breakfast: Banana Split Yogurt (See page 36)

Lunch: Greek Fish Tacos

Time: 25 minutes | Servings 6

Kcal 240, Carbs 24g/0.8oz, Proteins 25g/0.88oz, Fats 5g/0.18oz, Fiber 3g/0.11oz

INGREDIENTS

- 15ml/1 tablespoon of olive oil
- 250g/2 cups of shredded red or green cabbage
- 128g/1 cup of Kalamata olives halved
- 64g/½ cup of crumbled feta cheese
- Salt and pepper to taste
- 450g/1lb of firm white fish
- 1 cup of shredded red or green cabbage
- 128g/8 small soft flour or corn tortillas
- 128g/1 cup of grape or cherry tomatoes, thinly sliced
- 1 cucumber, seeded and diced
- Then finally, tzatziki sauce for the topping

PREPARATION

1. Season both sides of the fish with pinches of pepper and salt. Afterward, heat the oil in a saucepan over medium heat and cook them for about 5 minutes per side till it is cooked through. Remove the fish from the heat and then use a fork to flake the fish into small bite-sized pieces.

2. Assemble the tacos and then top with feta and the tzatziki to taste and then serve with lemon wedges for the squeeze of juice.

Dinner: Greek Stuffed Mushroom Portobellos (See page 53)

DAY 3

Breakfast: The Honey Almond Ricotta Spread with Fruit
Time: 5 minutes | Servings 6
Kcal 199, Carbs 13g/0.46oz, Proteins 8.5g/0.3oz, Fats 12g/0.42oz, Fiber 3g/0.11oz

INGREDIENTS

- 250ml/1 cup of whole milk
- 2ml/¼ teaspoon of almond extract
- 5ml/1 teaspoon of honey

- This is optional, but it is needed for a wholesome meal. The Zest from an orange
- 65g/½ cup of fisher sliced almonds

While for the serving, you should add:

- Extra honey for the drizzling
- Sliced peaches are also needed

- Whole grain toast, bagel, or English muffin
- You need some extra fisher almonds

PREPARATION

1. All you need to do is to combine the almonds, almond extract, ricotta in a suitable mixing bowl, and then stir gently to combine. This you should transfer to a serving bowl and then sprinkle with some more almonds and then drizzle with a teaspoon of honey.

2. To serve this delicacy, toast the bread and spread a teaspoon of ricotta spread on each slice. Then move to top with some more sliced almonds, peaches, and honey.

Lunch: Mediterranean Veggie Sandwich (See page 40)
Dinner: Mediterranean Ravioli with Artichokes and Olives (See page 54)

DAY 4

Breakfast: Breakfast Zucchini Noodles
Time: 20 minutes | Servings 4
Kcal 633, Fat 53g/2oz, Protein 20g/0.71oz, Sugars 9g/0.32oz, Carbs 27g/0.95oz

INGREDIENTS

- 4 eggs
- 2 avocados, halved and sliced thinly
- A non-stick spray
- 3 zucchinis, well spiralized into noodles
- 30ml/2 tablespoons of extra-virgin olive oil
- Red pepper flakes for garnishing
- Fresh basil for the garnishing
- Kosher salt with freshly ground black pepper

PREPARATION

1. As usual, preheat the oven to about 350F, then grease the baking sheet with the nonstick spray you have ready. In a large bowl combine the olive oil and zucchini noodles; after, season with pepper and salt. Move to divide into about four (4) portions and then transfer to a baking sheet while shaping each to look like a nest.

2. Crack the egg into the center of the nest like shape you have, bake until it is set for about 10 minutes. Season with pepper and salt, garnish with basil and red pepper flakes, and then serve with avocado slices.

Lunch: Falafel Kale Salad with the Best Tahini Dressing (See page 41)

Dinner: Prosciutto Pizza with Corn and Arugula (See page 55)

DAY 5

Breakfast: The Breakfast Hash with Brussels Sprouts
and Sweet Potatoes (See page 24)

Lunch: Salmon Souvlaki Bowls

Time: 25 minutes | Servings 3

Kcal 165, Carbs 14.4g/0.51oz, Protein 9g/0.32oz, Fat 9.2g/0.33oz, Fiber 3.8g/0.13oz

INGREDIENTS

- 90ml/6 tablespoons of lemon juice
- 45ml/3 tablespoons of olive oil
- 450g/1lb of fresh salmon fish cut into 4 pieces
- 30ml/2 tablespoons of balsamic vinegar
- 17g/1 tablespoon of fresh dill

- 17g/1 tablespoon of fresh oregano
- ½ cloves of garlic minced and grated
- 17g/1 tablespoon of pepper
- 2g/½ teaspoon of salt
- 4g/1 teaspoon of pepper

For the Bowls:

- 2 quartered red peppers
- 128g/1 cup of dry pearl couscous or even farro
- 128g/1 cup of cherry tomatoes halved
- 230g/8oz of feta cheese crumbled
- Juice from one lemon
- 2 sliced Persian cucumbers
- 30ml/2 tablespoons of olive oil

- 64g/½ cup of Kalamata olives
- 1-inch zucchini cut into ¼ rounds

PREPARATION

1. In a suitable bowl, combine the lemon juice, vinegar, smoked paprika, oregano, dill, garlic, pepper and salt, and olive oil. Add the salmon and toss very well, making sure the salmon is well coated in the seasonings. Cook the couscous or farro according to the instructions and in another separate bowl, combine the zucchini, olive oil, salt, red peppers, and all and also toss well to coat the veggies.

2. Heat the grill to medium heat and then transfer the salmon to the grill already preheated for some minutes until the salmon is done. Remove it and add the zucchini and bell peppers, grill for some minutes per side until the marks appear, and then remove everything from the grill. Assemble the farro or the couscous accordingly, add the veggies, and drizzle with olive oil. Top everything with the tzatziki sauce and garnish with some fresh herbs.

Dinner: Greek Burgers with Herb-Feta Sauce (See page 56)

DAY 6

Breakfast: Smoked Salmon and Poached Eggs on Toast
Time: 15 minutes | Servings 3
Kcal 190, Carbs 14g/0.49oz, Proteins 14g/0.49oz, Fats 8g/0.28oz, Fiber 3g/0.11oz

INGREDIENTS

- 17g/1 tablespoon of scallions sliced thinly
- Microgreens, although optional
- 2 slices of toasted bread
- ½ of a large avocado smashed
- 1g/¼ teaspoon of freshly squeezed lemon juice
- 2 poached eggs
- A pinch of cracked black pepper and kosher salt
- A splash of Kikkoman soy sauce

PREPARATION

1. In a suitable bowl, smash the avocado and then add lemon juice and a pinch of salt. Combine very well and then set it aside. Poach the eggs and when they are in an ice bath, proceed to toast the bread. After it is toasted, spread avocado on both the slices of bread and add smoked salmon to the slice.

2. Transfer the poached eggs to their toasts. And then hit all you have on the ground with a splash of the Kikkoman soy sauce and the cracked pepper. Garnish with microgreens and scallions.

Lunch: Mediterranean Quinoa Bowls with Roast-
ed Red Pepper Sauce (See page 42)

Dinner: Salmon Pita Sandwich (See page 57)

DAY 7

Breakfast: Avocado Tomato Gouda Socca Pizza (See page 29)

Lunch: Mediterranean Tuna Salad

Time: 5 minutes | Servings 2

Kcal 155, Fat 16g/0.56oz, Carbs 2g/0.07oz, Proteins 14g/0.49oz, Fiber 1g/0.03oz

INGREDIENTS

- 34g/2 tablespoons of capers
- 32g/¼ cup of roasted red peppers diced
- Salt and pepper to taste
- 30ml/2 tablespoons of olive oil
- 17g/1 tablespoon of chopped, fresh parsley
- 15ml/1 tablespoon of lemon juice
- 450g/1lb can selections of solid white albacore tuna, fully water drained

PREPARATION

1. Just add all the ingredients together in a mixing bowl and then make use of a fork to piece out the tuna and then mix. Serve almost immediately and you may also choose to refrigerate the leftovers.

   Dinner: Gluten-Free Pasta Mediterranean Style (See page 58)

DAY 8

Breakfast: Greek Yogurt Pancakes
Time: 15 minutes | Servings 4
Kcal 258, Fat 8g/0.28oz, Carbs 33g/1.16oz, Protein 11g/0.40oz, Fiber 1g/0.03oz

INGREDIENTS

- 8g/2 teaspoons of baking powder
- 4g/1 teaspoon of baking soda
- 3 eggs
- 375ml/1½ cups of Greek plain yogurt
- 125ml/½ cup of milk
- 64g/½ cup of blueberries which are optional depending on your discretion
- 200g/1¼ cup of an all-purpose flour
- 1g/¼ teaspoon of salt
- 32g/¼ cup of sugar
- 45ml/3 tablespoons of unsalted butter, and melted

PREPARATION

1. Whisk the flour, baking powder, baking soda, and salt in a bowl, then in a separate bowl proceed to also mix the butter, sugar, Greek yogurt, eggs, and milk until it is smooth. After this, add the Greek yogurt mixture from the second step to the mixture you made the first time and then mix well to properly combine.

2. After this, heat up the pancake griddle and then spray with a non-stick butter spray or you can just choose to brush the griddle with actual butter. Pour the batter you have made in quarter cups and onto the griddle. Then cook them until the bubbles form on top burst and create small holes. Then lift the corners of each pancake and then check if it is browned already at the bottom.

3. Then using a wide, suitable spatula in all, flip the pancake and cook until it is lightly browned. Remove the pancakes from the griddle to the warming plate and you can serve almost immediately.

Lunch: Greek Zucchini and Walnut Salad (See page 48)

Dinner: Mediterranean Stuffed Sweet Potatoes with Chickpeas and Avocado Tahini (See page 60)

DAY 9

Breakfast: Greek Omelet Casserole (See page 31)
Lunch: Beet and Winter Shrimp Salad (See page 47)
Dinner: The Spanish Garlic Shrimp
Time: 20 minutes | Servings 3
Kcal 250, Carbs 3.4g/0.12oz, Protein 15.8g/0.6oz, Fat 17.9g/0.63oz, Fiber 0.4g/0.0014oz

INGREDIENTS

- 4 cloves of finely chopped garlic
- 34g/2 tablespoons of chopped parsley
- 34g/2 tablespoons of dry sherry
- 1g/¼ teaspoon of kosher salt
- 80ml/⅓ cup of olive oil
- 1g/¼ teaspoon of chili flakes
- 450g/1lb of large shrimp, deveined and peeled
- 4g/1 teaspoon of sweet Spanish paprika
- A pinch of pepper
- 35ml/1½ tablespoons of fresh lemon juice

PREPARATION

1. Just pour the oil into a large pan and add the chili flakes and garlic. Turn up the heat a little and as it heats up, the oil will get infused slowly with the flavor of the chili and garlic. Once this has been left for some minutes, add the shrimp to the mixture, season with salt, pepper, and paprika. Cook the shrimp for some minutes until they turn pink.

2. Add the lemon juice and sherry at this point and then cook for some more minutes until when the liquid is reduced and the shrimp is properly cooked. Sprinkle the parsley on top and then serve with crusty bread, ideal for soaking up the sauce.

DAY 10

Breakfast: Banana Mocha Overnight Oats
Time: 8 hours 10 minutes | Servings 4
Kcal 283, Carbs 7g/0.25oz, Fats 18.9g/0.7oz, Proteins 16.5g/0.58oz, Fibers 8g/0.28oz

INGREDIENTS

- 125ml/½ a cup of strong coffee. The cold brew technique works well too
- 34g/2 tablespoons of cocoa powder
- 128g/1 cup of rolled oats
- 1 banana, as expected
- Fresh fruits of your choice for the serving
- 30g/1½ tablespoons of chia seeds
- 200ml/¾ cup of almond milk or any non-dairy milk of your choice. P.s, remember what we have been talking about the foods you can eat and those you cannot when on the Mediterranean diet.
- 2 dates, well pitted just in case your blender is not strong enough. As an alternative, you can decide to soak the dates in warm water for some time, and care to drain very well before blending.

1. All you have to do is to blend the almond milk, coffee, dates, cocoa powder, dates, sea salt, and banana in a blender and blend till it is very smooth. After this, place the chia seeds and oats in an airtight container. Then pour the liquid mixture over the chia seeds you have and then stir everything to combine properly.

2. Just cover and refrigerate well. In the morning take out your oats, stir it very well and then add a small splash of non-dairy milk and generously top with fresh fruit to enjoy it.

Lunch: Couscous and Chickpea Salad (See page 46)

Dinner: Slow-Cooker Mediterranean Stew (See page 51)

DAY 11

Breakfast: Cauliflower Fritters with Hummus (See page 32)
Lunch: The Mediterranean Vegan Salad (See page 49)
Dinner: The Quinoa Tabbouleh
Time: 22 minutes | Servings 2
Kcal 412, Carbs 74.5g/2.63oz, Protein 17.5g/0.62oz, Fiber 14.3g/0.5oz, Fat 6.5g/0.23oz

INGREDIENTS

- 500ml/2 cups of water
- 128g/1 cup of parsley finely chopped
- The juice of 1 lemon, and extra olive oil to taste
- 128g/1 cup of quinoa
- 128g/1 cup of freshly chopped parsley
- 160g/1⅓ cup of chopped tomatoes
- 64g/½ a cup of spring onions

PREPARATION

1. Simply move to rinse the quinoa with water, boil the water in a suitable saucepan and add the quinoa. Simmer for some minutes till all the water has been absorbed. You can also move to add the other you may have to the boiling water for more flavor.

2. Allow the quinoa to cool for some minutes at room temperature or you can choose to add cold water till it is cool enough to make the salad. Then in a large bowl, place the quinoa and the rest of the as mentioned earlier.

3. You can also add the extra virgin oil, and lemon juice, stir and serve almost immediately.

DAY 12

Breakfast: Avocado Toast with Persimmon, Fennel, and Pomegranate
Time: 10 minutes | Servings 2
Kcal 377, Carbs 41.6g/1.46oz, Fats 22.6g/0.8oz, Proteins 7.1g/0.25oz, Fiber 1g/0.03oz

INGREDIENTS

- 17g/1 tablespoon of goat cheese
- 1g/¼ teaspoon of salt
- 3ml/½ teaspoon of lime juice
- 1 avocado
- Persimmon, thinly sliced

- 34g/2 tablespoons of pomegranate seeds
- 10ml/2 teaspoon of honey
- Fennel bulb, thinly sliced with a few fennel fronds
- 2 pieces of bread, already toasted

PREPARATION

1. This is also another breakfast meal you can prepare within minutes. All you have to do is to cut the avocado into half and scoop out the flesh into a bowl. Afterward, add the lime juice, salt, and goat cheese and then mash lightly with a fork.

2. Move to spread the mashed avocado you have onto the toasted bread, taking care to divide it evenly between the two slices. After this, top with some slices of fennel and persimmon. Then sprinkle with pomegranate seeds and fennel fronds. Drizzle all with honey and then proceed to serve.

Lunch: The Classic Mediterranean Salad (See page 39)
Dinner: Casserole Fish with Mushroom and French Mustard (See page 62)

DAY 13

Breakfast: Greek Salad Sushi (See page 34)

Lunch: Mediterranean Veggie Sandwich (See page 40)

Dinner: Walnut Rosemary Crusted Salmon

Time: 20 minutes | Servings 4

Kcal 222, Fat 12g/0.42oz, Protein 24g/0.85oz, Carbohydrates 4g/0.14oz, Fiber 1g/0.04oz

INGREDIENTS

- 1 clove of garlic
- 8g/2 teaspoons of Dijon mustard
- 4g/1 teaspoon of chopped, fresh, good quality rosemary
- 2g/½ teaspoon of kosher salt
- 2g/½ teaspoon of honey
- 4g/1 teaspoon of lemon juice
- 1g/¼ teaspoon of lemon zest
- 51g/3 tablespoons of panko breadcrumbs
- 5ml/1 teaspoon of extra virgin olive oil
- 1g/¼ teaspoon of crushed red pepper
- 450g/1lb of skinless salmon, fresh or frozen
- Nicely chopped fresh parsley and lemon wedges for the garnish

PREPARATION

1. First, preheat the oven to around 425 degrees and also line the baking sheet with parchment paper. After this, combine the lemon zest, juice, honey, salt, rosemary, mustard, garlic, and crushed red pepper in a small bowl. Then combine the walnuts, oil, and panko breadcrumbs in another small bowl.

2. Move to place the salmon on the baking sheet you have already prepared and then spread the mustard mixture all over the fish and also sprinkle some on the panko mixture, while pressing it to make sure it adheres. Coat lightly with the cooking spray you have.

3. After all, is said and done, bake until all the fish is soft enough. This can be for about 8 to 10 minutes depending on the thickness of the fish. Then sprinkle with the fresh parsley and serve with wedges of lemon, depending on what you enjoy.

DAY 14

Breakfast: Mediterranean Breakfast Salad
Time: 20 minutes | Servings 4
Kcal 145, Carbs 2g/0.06oz, Fats 14g/0.49oz, Proteins 1g/0.03oz, Fiber 1g/0.03oz

INGREDIENTS

- ½ seedless cucumber, properly chopped
- 1 large avocado
- 4 eggs
- 1289g/10 cups of arugula
- 128g/1 cup of cooked quinoa, properly cooled
- 1 lemon
- Extra virgin olive oil
- Sea salt and black pepper, freshly ground
- 64g/½ a cup of mixed herbs like dill and mint, chopped
- 250g/2 cups of halved cherry tomatoes or heirloom tomatoes even

PREPARATION

1. The eggs are the first you would cook. Boil in water for some minutes, but do note that the minutes may vary based on the type of egg you want. Soft boiled or not. After this, lower the eggs into the water gently and allow cold water to run over it to stop the cooking. Set it aside and peel when you are ready to make use of it.

2. Combine tomatoes, cucumber, quinoa, and arugula in a large bowl. After, drizzle a little olive oil over the top of all you have down, and then season to taste with salt and pepper, then toss all of it together.

3. Finally, divide the salad into 4 plates. Then top with halved egg and sliced avocado. Sprinkle the herbs and almonds over the top and then season some more with salt and pepper. Add a squeeze of lemon juice and drizzle of olive oil. Your salad is ready!!

Lunch: Falafel Kale Salad with the Best Tahini Dressing (See page 41)

Dinner: Mediterranean Ravioli with Artichokes and Olives (See page 54)

DAY 15

Breakfast: Greek Salad Sushi (See page 34)

*Lunch: Mediterranean Quinoa Bowls with Roast-
ed Red Pepper Sauce (See page 42)*

Dinner: Mediterranean Chicken and Barley Salad

Time: 30 minutes | Servings 2

Kcal 259, Carbs 23g/0.8oz, Fats 10.5g/0.37oz, Proteins 23g/0.8oz, Fiber 6g/0.21oz

INGREDIENTS

For the Barley:

- 375ml/1½ cups of water
- A pinch of salt
- 64g/½ a cup of barley spelt mixture or barley itself

For the Salad:

- 3 small cucumbers, well diced
- 2 tomatoes, diced and seeded
- ½ tsp of sumac
- 17g/1 tablespoon of lemon zest
- 2 cooked boneless, skinless, chicken breasts, shredded
- 51g/3 tablespoons of crumbled and reduced feta cheese
- 5 tomatoes, sundried, rehydrated, and minced
- 30ml/2 tablespoons of olive oil
- 51g/3 tablespoons of sunflower seeds
- Salt to taste
- 34g/2 tablespoons of mint chiffonade
- 2g/½ teaspoon of red pepper flakes
- The juice of ½ of a lemon

PREPARATION

1. This is easy to prepare, put the barley spelt mixture you have, a pinch of salt, water in a suitable saucepot and boil. Then reduce the heat to a medium-low and continue to simmer for about 15minutes till the water has absorbed. You can now remove from the heat and cool.

2. In another large bowl, mix all the veggies, the chicken, the lemon juice, red pepper flakes, mint, salt, sunflower seeds and all. After doing all this, divide them in equal proportions and enjoy them.

DAY 16

Breakfast: Muesli with Raspberries (See page 35)
Lunch: Lemon and Parmesan Chicken with Zucchini Noodles (See page 43)
Dinner: Mediterranean Fig and Mozzarella Salad
Time: 5 minutes | Servings 2

Kcal 286, Carbs 11g/0.38oz, Protein 10g/0.35oz, Fats 9g/0.317oz, Fiber 3g/0.105oz

INGREDIENTS

- 6 small, quartered figs
- 50g/1.8oz hazelnut, chopped and toasted
- 15ml/1 tablespoon fig jam or relish
- 45ml/3 tablespoons of extra virgin olive oil
- 200g/7.05oz of green bean, trimmed
- 45ml/3 tablespoon of balsamic vinegar
- Torn, small basil leaves
- 1 shallot, sliced thinly with a ball of mozzarella, ripped into chunks, and also drained

PREPARATION

1. The first step to preparing this is to blanch the beans for about 3 minutes. Drain the beans and rinse in cold water and then drain it out on kitchen paper. After doing this, arrange on a platter and then top with shallots, hazelnuts, basil, and mozzarella.

2. Making use of a small bowl or a jar of jam with a fitted lid, add the fig jam, olive oil, vinegar, and some seasoning. Shake it very well and then pour the salad over it before serving.

DAY 17

*Breakfast: The Breakfast Hash with Brussels Sprouts
and Sweet Potatoes (See page 24)*

Lunch: The Lemony Orzo Salad (See page 45)

Dinner: Mussels with Tomatoes and Chili

Time: 25 minutes | Servings 2

Kcal 267, Protein 20g/0.71oz, Fat 14g/0.49oz, Carbs 11g/0.38oz, Fiber 1g/0.04oz

INGREDIENTS

- 30ml/2 tablespoons of olive oil
- 5ml/1 teaspoon of tomato paste
- Handful basil leaves
- Pinch of sugar
- 2 ripe tomatoes
- 30ml/2 tablespoons of olive oil
- 1 finely chopped shallot
- 1 green or red chili, finely chopped and deseeded
- 1kg of clean mussels

PREPARATION

1. First put the tomatoes in a heatproof bowl, cover the boiling water and leave for some minutes. Drain and peel them; after this, quarter the tomatoes and then scoop out its contents and discard the seeds making use of a teaspoon. You can roughly cut the tomato flesh.

2. Heat oil in a suitable pan; add shallot, garlic, and chili. Fry gently for some minutes until it has softened and then pour in the wine and add the remaining veggies with sugar, seasoning, and paste. Stir the mixture very well and allow it to simmer for about 2 minutes.

3. Lastly, toss the mussels in and stir them. Steam and tightly cover for some minutes by shaking the pan, just until the shells have opened. Then discard any of the shells lying around remaining shut and then divide the basil leaves and divide the mussels between two similar-sized bowls. You can also provide a bowl for the empty leaves.

DAY 18

Breakfast: Mediterranean Egg Cups with Goat Cheese
Time: 40 minutes | Servings 6
Kcal 168, Carbs 5.1g/0.18oz, Fats 20.8g/0.73oz, Proteins 9.8g/0.35oz, Fiber 11g/0.38oz

INGREDIENTS

- 10 eggs
- 90g/⅔ cup of plain almond milk
- Olive oil or coconut spray
- 2g/½ teaspoon of garlic powder
- A pinch of salt
- 1g/¼ teaspoon of black pepper
- 190g/1½ cups of roasted bell peppers, rinsed, well-drained and any excess liquid blotted with a paper towel or a clean towel
- 190g/1½ cups of chopped mushrooms

PREPARATION

1. As usual, preheat your oven to around 350 degrees and then prepare a 12 cup muffin tin by only spraying it with a cooking spray, and still making sure you still spray the top with spray too just in case it goes over a bit. After doing all this, in a large bowl, mix the almond milk, garlic powder, salt and black pepper until you have the right consistency. Then also, remember to add the mushrooms and roasted peppers. Then move to fill each muffin cup with the mixture you just prepared.

2. Bake for about 30 minutes or until it is set. After this, remove from the oven and then allow the cakes cool in the pan for about 10 minutes so they will deflate a bit so they can be easily removed from the muffin tin. Then serve with some goat cheese and crumbles, all for garnishing.

Lunch: Couscous and Chickpea Salad (See page 46)

Dinner: Mediterranean Ravioli with Artichokes and Olives (See page 54)

DAY 19

Breakfast: Shak Shuka with Tofu 'FETA' (See page 26)
Lunch: Beet and Winter Shrimp Salad (See page 47)
Dinner: Mediterranean White Bean Salad
Time: 15 minutes | Servings 4

Kcal 210, Carbs 22g/0.78oz, Proteins 8.48g/0.3oz, Fats 9.08g/0.32oz, Fiber 7.28g/0.26oz

INGREDIENTS

- 1 cup pesto
- 17ml/1 tablespoon and 17ml/1 tablespoon of kosher salt
- 17ml/1 tablespoon of black pepper
- 425g/15oz of cannellini beans
- 5 stalks of celery, sliced
- Medium red bell pepper, well minced
- 50ml/1½oz of red wine vinegar
- 17g/1 tablespoon of black pepper

PREPARATION

1. This is simple to prepare; just drain the beans in a colander and rinse subsequently with cold water. Then set it aside to drain. In a large bowl, combine all the remaining and toss together very well.

DAY 20

Breakfast: Muesli with Raspberries

Time: 45 minutes | Servings 4

Kcal 295, Carbs 29.8g/1.05oz, Fats 13.4g/0.47oz, Proteins 13.7g/0.48oz, Fiber 5g/0.98oz

INGREDIENTS

- 15ml/1 tablespoon of olive oil or unsalted butter
- Freshly ground pepper added to taste
- 1g/¼ teaspoon of salt
- 750ml/3 cups of water
- 250ml/1 cup of neutral-flavored milk of your choice and an additional cup of water

PREPARATION

1. Mix water and milk in a bowl, in a suitable saucepan, and then place on medium heat to allow it to simmer. While doing this, melt the butter or warm the olive oil in an appropriately sized skillet also on medium heat. After the period of sizzling has elapsed, add the oats, reduce the heat a bit and then simmer gently while stirring continuously, until you have a thick mixture.

2. Proceed to stir in the salt, continue to simmer, and reduce the heat to prevent the bottom of the pot from scorching. You can decide to wait till almost half of the entire mixture is absorbed. Although it is possible the oatmeal takes some time to cook, be assured it will be very creamy when done.

3. Remove entirely from the heat and allow the oatmeal to rest for some minutes before you serve; this is to allow the mixture to thicken up and then cool it down to a reasonable temperature. Season it generously with salt and enough pepper.

4. Divide the oatmeal into different portions; garnish with any toppings you might like and let the extra oatmeal cool down very completely before it is refrigerated and completely cover it too; this may look simple, but it is highly essential.

Lunch: The Classic Mediterranean Salad (See page 39)

Dinner: Prosciutto Pizza with Corn and Arugula (See page 55)

DAY 21

Breakfast: Mediterranean Diet Scrambled Eggs (See page 28)

Lunch: Mediterranean Veggie Sandwich (See page 40)

Dinner: Easy Chicken Piccata

Time: 30 minutes | Servings 3

Kcal 232, Carbs 6.4g/0.22oz, Fats 19g/0.67oz, Protein 8.5g/0.3oz, Fiber 3.8g/0.13oz

INGREDIENTS

- 4g/1 teaspoon of kosher salt
- 1 lemon
- 4g/1 teaspoon of freshly ground black pepper
- 30ml/2 tablespoons of canola oil
- 250ml/1 cup of chicken broth or white wine or even a combination of both may be ideal
- 30ml/2 tablespoons of capers drained and rinsed
- 680g/1½lb of skinless, boneless chicken breasts
- 40g/⅓ cup of an all-purpose flour
- 34g/2 tablespoons of capers rinsed and drained

PREPARATION

1. The first thing to do is to slice the lemon in half, juice one half, and cut the other in different slices and then set it aside. Trim off any excess fat off the chicken breasts you have and slice in half. Season both sides of the chicken breasts evenly and the kosher salt and ground pepper respectively. Dredge each of the breasts in flour and shake off any excess.

2. Heat the tablespoon of butter you have, with the canola oil in a large skillet over medium heat and then add about 4 pieces of chicken and cook for some minutes per side. Transfer to a sheet pan and cover the foil, continue with the rest of the chicken.

3. Reduce the heat to medium or as desired and add the wine or chicken broth, the lemons, its juice, and the capers. Scrape the browned bits off the pan and cook for about 3 minutes. Stir in the remaining tablespoon of butter until it is melted. Taste the seasoning and see if enough and then spoon some over the chicken breasts. Your meal is ready and you can choose to serve it with noodles, polenta, or mashed potatoes.

DAY 22

Breakfast: Avocado Tomato Gouda Socca Pizza (See page 29)

Lunch: 30 Minute Shrimp Grain Bowls

Time: 30 minutes | Servings 4

Kcal 239, Fats 7.1g/0.25oz, Carbs 19g/0.67oz, Protein 24.8g/0.87oz, Fiber 2.3g/0.081oz

INGREDIENTS

- 30ml/2 tablespoons of fresh lemon juice
- 2 cloves of garlic, properly minced
- 65ml/¼ cup of extra virgin olive oil
- 17g/1 teaspoon of dried oregano
- 128g/1 cup of dry farro or even white rice
- 500ml/2 cups of vegetable or chicken broth
- 4g/1 teaspoon of smoked paprika

- 5g/¾ teaspoon of kosher salt
- 2 small zucchinis. Sliced into coins
- 450g/1lb of deveined and peeled shrimp
- 2g/½ teaspoon of black pepper
- 2 bell peppers sliced into small pieces
- The optional garnishes include cherry tomatoes, capers, sliced green olives

Lemon-Garlic Yogurt:

- 1 garlic clove, properly grated
- 1g/¼ teaspoon of kosher salt
- 15ml/1 tablespoon of lemon juice
- 125ml/½ cup of plain Greek yogurt

PREPARATION

1. Combine the first seven earlier outlined in a suitable bowl and whisk properly. Place the vegetables and shrimps in separate bowls and then divide and marinade evenly. After this, allow it to stand for about 10 minutes.

2. Combine the farro or rice depending on the one available in a saucepan with the broth. Boil, and then reduce the heat to low and simmer gently until the grains are tender and most of the liquid is absorbed.

3. In the meantime, heat a large skillet properly coated in a cooking spray overheat adjusted to medium-high. Once it is hot, add the shrimp and then cook for 2 minutes per side until it is opaque. Then transfer to a plate, add the vegetables to the skillet and cook until it is tender, just for about 8 minutes.

4. Prepare the lemon garlic yogurt by combining the garlic, lemon juice, and salt in a suitable bowl. Stir in little water to achieve the desired consistency. Assemble all the bowls by dividing rice or farro into each of the 4 bowls you might have set out. Scatter the vegetables and shrimp on top and finish with the lemon-garlic yogurt. Based on your discretion, you might decide to garnish generously with olives, fresh herbs, and cherry tomatoes with a drizzle of olive oil.

Dinner: Greek Burgers with Herb-Feta Sauce (See page 56)

DAY 23

Breakfast: Greek Omelet Casserole (See page 31)
Lunch: Bulgur Salad with Marinated Feta
Time: 12 hours 10 minute | Servings 4
Kcal 233, Carbs 2.9g/0.1oz, Fats 5.6g/0.19oz, Proteins 5.8g/0.2oz, Fiber 1g/0.03oz

INGREDIENTS

For Marinated Feta:

- 5g/1 teaspoon of lemon zest
- 60ml/½ cup feta, cut into halves
- 4g/1 teaspoon of finely chopped fresh oregano leaves

- 4g/1 teaspoon of coarsely ground black pepper
- Olive oil
- 2g/½ teaspoon of garlic powder

For the Bulgur Salad:

- 375ml/1½ cup of boiling water
- 60ml/¼ cup of minced fresh parsley
- 1 cucumber, with seeds already removed with a spoon and diced properly
- 60g/½ cup of diced tomato
- 128g/1 cup of bulgur wheat
- 32g/¼ cup of minced fresh mint leaves
- 30ml/2 tablespoons of lemon juice
- Salt

- Whole mint leaves to garnish

PREPARATION

1. For the marinated feta, place the feta in a suitable bowl and then add oregano and lemon zest; season with black pepper and garlic powder. Transfer the mixture you have to a jar or a Tupperware with a lid. Then proceed to cover the cheese with olive oil and then cover the container and refrigerate for at least 12 hours.

2. For the bulgur salad, place the bulgur in a bowl and cover with boiling water. Stir it quickly and allow it to sit at about the room temperature for some minutes until it has softened slightly. Strain it of any liquid that may be remaining.

3. Then mix in the chopped tomato, lemon juice, parsley, mint, chopped cucumber, and then season it all with salt to taste. And serve almost immediately with marinated feta.

Dinner: Roasted Vegetable Mediterranean (See page 63)

DAY 24

Breakfast: Cauliflower Fritters with Hummus (See page 32)

Lunch: Hummus and Greek Salad

Time: 5 minutes | Servings 3

Kcal 422, Fat 29.9g/1.05oz, Carbs 30.5g/1.07oz, Protein 10.9g/0.38oz, Sugar 4g/0.141oz

INGREDIENTS

- 40g/⅓ cup of cherry tomatoes, and halved
- 40g/⅓ cup of sliced cucumber
- 250g/2 cups of arugula
- 17g/1 tablespoon of chopped red onion
- 8g/2 teaspoons of red wine vinegar
- 17g/1 tablespoon of feta cheese
- 25ml/1½ tablespoons of extra virgin olive oil
- A pinch of grounded pepper
- 32g/¼ cup of hummus
- 1 4-inch of whole wheat pita

PREPARATION

1. It is simple to prepare. Just toss the arugula in a bowl with onions, cucumbers, oil, onion, pepper and vinegar, and tomatoes. Top with feta and serve with hummus and pita.

Dinner: Gluten-Free Pasta Mediterranean Style (See page 58)

DAY 25

Breakfast: Greek Salad Sushi (See page 34)

Lunch: Israeli Pasta Salad

Time: 20 minutes | Servings 2

Kcal 401, Carbs 64g/2.25oz, Fats 10g/0.3oz, Proteins 15g/0.53oz, Fiber 12g/0.42oz

INGREDIENTS

- 40g/⅓ cup of finely diced radish
- 40g/⅓ cup of finely diced orange pepper
- 40g/⅓ cup of green olives, finely diced
- 40g/⅓ cup of finely diced feta cheese
- 40g/⅓ cup of pepperoncini diced
- 275g/½lb of small bow tie or any other small pasta
- 40g/⅓ cup of cucumber, finely diced
- 40g/⅓ cup of tomato, finely diced
- 40g/⅓ cup of yellow bell pepper, also diced
- 4g/1 teaspoon of dried oregano
- Salt and fresh cracked black pepper to taste
- Fresh thyme leaves

PREPARATION

1. Cook the pasta you have very well in properly salted water until it is just al dente. Make sure you do not overcook and also drain and rinse in cold water after. Put the pasta in a suitable bowl and drizzle with olive oil so it does not stick. Then add the thyme, salt, pepper, veggies, and thyme. Make sure you hold out on the feta cheese till the end.

2. Add the olive oil you have and lemon juice as well and toss very well. Then gently fold in the feta cheese. Before enjoying the salad for a minimum of at least 2 hours or even overnight. Taste before you serve as you might want to add more lemon, salt, and olive oil or pepper based on your taste buds.

3. After all is said and done, garnish all with fresh thyme.

Dinner: Mediterranean Stuffed Sweet Potatoes with Chickpeas and Avocado Tahini (See page 60)

DAY 26

Breakfast: Muesli with Raspberries (See page 35)

Lunch: Greek Turkey Meatball Gyro with Tzatziki

Time: 15 minutes | Servings 4

Kcal 429, Carbs 38g/1.34oz, Protein 28g/0.98oz, Fat 19g/0.67oz, Fiber 3g/0.105oz

INGREDIENTS

- 2 garlic cloves, minced.
- 32g/¼ cup of finely diced red onion
- 450g/1lb ground turkey
- 4g/1 teaspoon oregano

For the Tzatziki Sauce:

- 2g/½ teaspoon of dry dill
- Salt to taste
- 128g/1 cup of diced cucumber
- 128g/1 cup of diced tomato
- 4 wheat flatbreads
- 125ml/½ cup of plain Greek yogurt
- 32g/¼ cup of grated cucumber
- 3ml/2 tablespoons of lemon juice
- 64g/½ cup of thinly sliced red onion

- Salt and pepper to season
- 30ml/2 tablespoons of olive oil
- 128g/1 cup of fresh and chopped spinach

PREPARATION

1. In a suitable bowl add the diced onions, minced garlic, fresh spinach, pepper and salt, ground turkey and make good use of your hands, mix all the till the meat forms a ball, and sticks together. Then also using your hands, form the meat mixture into balls.

2. Heat a suitable skillet to mildly high heat; add olive oil and then add the meatballs. Cook each side for about 5 minutes till all the sides are all equally browned. Then remove from the pan and allow it to rest.

3. After this, in a small bowl add the Greek yogurt, lemon juice, dill, garlic powder, cucumber, and salt to taste. Then mix it till it is combined. Assemble the gyros by adding them to a flatbread, add sliced onions, cucumber, and tomato and then top with tzatziki sauce and your meal is ready.

Dinner: Slow-Cooker Mediterranean Stew (See page 51)

DAY 27

Breakfast: Quick and Easy Greek Salad (See page 37)
Lunch: Mediterranean Bento
Time: 5 minutes | Servings 2
Kcal 497, Fat 13.8g/0.48oz, Carbs 60.5g/2.13oz, Protein 36.7g/1.29oz, Fiber 7.9g/0.28oz

INGREDIENTS

- 32g/¼ cup of diced tomato
- 17g/1 tablespoon of diced olives
- 32g/¼ cup of chickpeas, rinsed
- 32g/¼ cup of cucumber
- 17g/1 tablespoon of crumbled feta cheese
- 4g/1 teaspoon of red wine vinegar
- 17g/1 tablespoon of chopped fresh parsley
- 2g/½ teaspoon of red wine vinegar
- 85g/3oz of grilled turkey breast tenderloin or chicken breast
- 128g/1 cup of grapes
- 34g/2 tablespoons of hummus
- 1 whole-wheat pita bread, and quartered

PREPARATION

1. Gather the cucumber, tomato, olives, feta, parsley, vinegar, feta, chickpeas, in a suitable bowl, and then pack in a medium-sized container. Pack the turkey or chicken in a medium container and lastly, pack the pita and grapes in small containers and the hummus in a dip size container.

   Dinner: Greek Stuffed Mushroom Portobellos (See page 53)

DAY 28

Breakfast: Shak Shuka with Tofu 'FETA' (See page 26)

Lunch: Vegan Smoky Moussaka

Time: 60 minutes | Servings 4

Kcal 341, Carbs 36g/1.27oz, Protein 16g/0.56oz, Fat 17g/0.59oz, Fiber 14g/0.49oz

INGREDIENTS

- 🍽 17g/1 tablespoon of tomato paste
- 🍽 2 onions, thinly sliced
- 🍽 5ml/1 teaspoon of maple syrup
- 🍽 1 can of plum tomatoes
- 🍽 A pinch of cinnamon

- 🍽 A pinch of cayenne pepper
- 🍽 A pinch of ground black pepper
- 🍽 340g/12oz of smoked tofu
- 🍽 2 cloves of garlic, properly chopped

For Eggplant:

- 🍽 15ml/1 tablespoon of olive oil, and 3 medium eggplants

Béchamel:

- 🍽 750ml/2½ cups of almond milk
- 🍽 2g/½ teaspoon of salt
- 🍽 A pinch of ground nutmeg
- 🍽 34g/2 tablespoon of nutritional yeast
- 🍽 34g/2 tablespoon of potato starch

1. Firstly, drain all the tomatoes in a bowl and keep the juice. Cut the plum tomatoes available into small pieces and then add them to a skillet with the juice. Heat them over medium heat, and be patient enough till the sauce thickens. Say for about ten minutes.

2. Stir in the maple syrup, salt, pepper, cinnamon, tomato paste, and then remove from the heat. Proceed to wash and cut the eggplants into about one-inch-thick slices, coupled with olive oil, and sprinkle with salt. Fry these slices till they turn tender and golden brown on both sides in a non-stick skillet over medium heat.

3. Transfer the eggplant slices to paper towels and then heat one tablespoon of olive oil over medium heat. Add garlic and onions and then cook until it is soft. Just for about 7 minutes. After this, move to scramble the smoked tofu and add this to the skillet. Cook it for some minutes, while stirring every 2 minutes. Add the tomato sauce you have and mix it till it is all combined and then remove from the heat.

4. Preheat the oven to around 400 degrees as usual. Arrange a layer of half the slices of eggplant in a fully greased baking dish. Cover with the tofu/tomato sauce and then top with another layer of eggplant slices. After this, pour the béchamel over the top and spread so it is even. Bake all for about 30 minutes, until the top turns golden brown and then top with chopped parsley.

For Béchamel:

To prepare the béchamel, add the ½ cup of almond milk to a medium-sized saucepan. Mix in the nutritional yeast, potato starch, nutmeg, and salt. Whisk everything until it is well combined and then add the remaining milk. Then heat all over medium heat for some minutes; whisk constantly until it thickens and then remove them from heat.

Dinner: Casserole Fish with Mushroom and French Mustard (See page 62)

Printed in Great Britain
by Amazon